HOW TO

CURE

Crohn's Disease

In

90 Days

Alternative Healthy Treatment
That Works

Table of Contents

Introduction

You're probably reading this book because you were diagnosed with Crohn's Disease! With this terrible disease, you're likely tired of the toilet being your best friend. You're sick and tired of all the meds you've been taking and they are not working for you anymore, and now you want a solution. Well guess what? That's why your reading this book! Because you want to change your health and how you feel on a daily basis. You're totally sick of being sick. Well, I can relate to many of these issues. And that's why I decided to take my health into my owns hands to find what was going to cure me. Because I certainly knew that if I left myself in the hands of my doctors, I would still be suffering today.

That word "cure" seems to be a very taboo word in the medical clinic and even on online forums and Crohn's Disease communities. I personally love the word and don't believe in the word remission. When you're in remission you still have an inflamed colon, but you're temporarily symptom free. What we want is to be fully healed with no inflammation in the colon so we don't get flare-ups and can eat what we want, right?

When you finish reading this book, you will also realize that you are not alone. You might also want to take the same path to healing your condition in 90-days as I did and so many others have also done, not leaving their destinies in the hands of the drug companies and doctors. I was just tired of seeing the gastrologist to change my meds every few months and yet my health never changed for the better. So I took action. Now that's what you need to do as well; to take your health by the throat and don't let go, until you're healthy again. It won't be an easy journey for you by any means. Not only will you need to have a tremendous amount of self-belief that you will get well, but it is physically and emotionally draining as well. You might find yourself getting worse before you get better. That's very important to keep in mind, but that's part of the healing process. This is not an easy program to follow. This is not an easy condition to cure and by no means does it happen overnight. It takes time and it's a very slow process, but if you follow everything in my guidelines you should be on your way to being healed within 90 days. At the very least, you will be in a remissive state give or take. However, some people do take a somewhat longer time frame and some will see great results in shorter time frame. It is very important (and I cannot emphasize this enough) that if you do not follow everything that is outlined in this book as far as what you need to take and how you need to eat do not expect to get good results to achieve total health with your condition to cure Crohn's Disease. You will need to follow everything precisely, so make sure that you go out and get everything you need before you start.

Why 90 days? The body is a very complex mechanism with many bio complex chemical electrical reactions going on all the time at a cellular level. Therefore the complexity of healing is present also. Meaning what? We need to provide the body with the correct nutrients so the body has the raw materials to keep those micro level bio electric functions in a healthy state and able to its job fighting disease in the body. Now keep in mind that we are all very diverse from one to another, some will see results sooner and others could take much longer, but be patient with your healing journey. Keep a day to day journal and reflect on what you ate that day: what supplements you took and how your body reacted. This will also help tremendously in your journey, but take it day by day. Plan on huge improvements on a weekly basis, stay positive and don't give up on your 90 day healing journey as we must not expect to see results over night when we have a chronic condition. Inflammation in the body takes time to heal. However, it took me 90 days to bring this condition to a point that I felt completely healthy, normal, and symptom free, living a normal life again, and you will too, along with hundreds of people who tried this protocol who have also had great success within the first 90 days.

****Before starting any program in this book it is advised to check with your personal physician first*****

"Time and health are two precious assets that we don't recognize and appreciate until they have been depleted"

Denis Waitley

1- What is Crohn's Disease

Crohn's Disease is a form of inflammatory bowel disease that is defined by chronic inflammation. This inflammation leads to the formation of ulcers in the colon primarily centralized in the small intestine but sometimes can include the large intestine and even the throat. The symptoms of Crohn's Disease include abdominal cramps, bloody diarrhea or diarrhea with pain and mucus. Other symptoms can include a great urge to defecate but being unable to do so, unexplained weight loss, tiredness, anemia, loss of appetite and fever. Crohn's disease usually spreads deep into the layers of the affected intestinal tissue. Crohn's disease is very debilitating, and can or may even lead to life-threatening complications. The severity and the type of symptoms depend on the severity of inflammation or what chronic stage the disease has achieved. According to the traditional medicine, they claim there is no known cure for Crohn's Disease; however with natural therapies, one can substantially reduce its signs and symptoms and even cure Crohn's.

With treatment, many people with Crohn's disease are able to function well and get back to a normal life again. You can likely relate to having some or all of these symptoms. Your symptoms may also vary during the course of your condition. Treatment for Crohn's Disease is usually medication or surgery.

Traditional medical treatment depends on the type and severity of Crohn's Disease. Sometimes people may experience more than one form or type of the disease at the same time. This means several areas of the digestive tract may be affected at one time. There are five types of Crohn's disease, each associated with its very specific symptoms and specific locations in the digestive tract, the following are the five different types of the disease:

- Ileocolitis
- Ileitis
- Gastroduodenal Crohn's disease
- Jejunoileitis
- Crohn's Colitis

Ileocolitis: Being the most common form of Crohn's Disease, most people diagnosed will suffer from Ileocolitis. This type of Crohn's Disease causes inflammation and major irritation of the ileum (the lower area of the small intestine). Those with Ileocolitis will experience following symptoms:

- Diarrhea
- Significant weight loss
- Pain, cramping in the middle area or the lower-right region of the abdomen

Ileitis: Like Ileocolitis, ileitis causes inflammation and also irritation of the ileum. The symptoms for ileitis are really the same as those for having Ileocolitis. Patients with ileitis may also develop fistulas (inflammatory abscesses) in the lower-right section of the abdomen.

Jejunoileitis: Develops in the jejunum, or the secondary part of the small intestine, these areas also get inflamed. Those diagnosed with Jejunoileitis may experience the following symptoms:

- Cramps after meals
- Fistulas
- Diarrhea
- Abdominal discomfort that can sometimes be severe

Gastroduodenal Crohn's Disease: Involves mostly the stomach and duodenum (leading part of the small intestine).People with this type of Crohn's disease will often experience nausea, weight loss, and lack of appetite. Those with gastroduodenal Crohn's disease may experience vomiting if parts of the bowel become blocked. This is all due to intestinal inflammation.

Crohn's (Granulomatous) Colitis: This type of Crohn's disease affects the parts of colon, which is the main area of the large intestine. It may cause ulcers, abscesses and fistulas that form around the anus. It can also cause the following symptoms:

- Skin lesions
- Joint pain
- Diarrhea
- Rectal bleeding

Now let's look at some statistics.

Canadians have even more reasons to be concerned about Crohn's Disease than other people. It's known that 20 cases per 100,000 people in Canada are living with Crohn's Disease. This is a statistic that is shockingly high when compared with numbers around the world. Families new to Canada are now developing Crohn's for the very first time. The number of new cases of Crohn's Disease in Canadian children has almost doubled since 1995

In the United States, Crohn's affects an estimated 1.4 Million people; it is the cause of 57,000 hospitalizations each year. There was an increase of doctors' visits from 1992 to 2004 of about 74 percent around the globe, and 141 million was spent on prescription drugs for the treatment of Crohn's Disease. Studies have reported an annual incidence of Crohn's ranging from 0.7 to 28.5 cases per 100,000 people. The disease affects an equal number of men and women. Crohn's is more common in Northern Europe and North America, although the rate of the disease in these areas has remained stable over the past fifty years. However, incidence has been rising in Asian and Southern European countries.

Let's take a look at how the medical community looks at this condition. The medical community classifies it in this dark hole of the incurables. They claim that there is not cure for this dreaded disease; they don't seem to know how it starts and certainly don't know how to put an end to it. Now how can we possibly believe that, when the human body has been designed by our Creator to heal all illnesses and disease in the body? The medical community has these ignorant claims, just as they claim there is no cure for cancer when thousands of people have cured their bodies of the incurable diseases. Healing is possible just with providing the natural raw resources, materials, minerals, vitamins and herbs that heal the body, cure the illness and not just mask the symptoms like the harsh traditional medications do.

"Health is not valued till sickness comes"

Thomas Fuller

2-Immune disorder or intestinal disorder?

The medical community seems to have to no real idea of how this disease manifests itself, how it starts what causes it, and why.

A gastrologist or your general practitioner will normally tell you the words you don't want to hear: There is no cure for this disease and that you are stuck with it for the rest of your life. Let me tell you right now, do not let their discouraging words bring your motivation down to battle this disease. They are simply following what they have been indoctrinated in and they are just following there medical protocol.

The medical community has some understanding that there is an Immunologic disorder factor involved and an intestinal microbiota out of balance that contributes to the inflammation in typical cases of Crohn's Disease patients. In part, I think they have studied what is gone wrong in the body in its current state of inflammation, but they have not figured out the cause of how it got to this state of extreme inflammation and deterioration of the colon.

In my studies and working with many people with Crohn's over the last 12 years, I have come to the conclusion that this disease manifests itself in different ways with different individuals. In some cases it has a more of a prevalent role with the immune system and others it has a stronger impact on an individual's microbiota in their colon. There is always some degree of influence on both at all times. Let me explain! If your disease is at a later stage or several years into it, the disease tends to have a bigger relation to an over active immunity instead of just an imbalance of microbus in your colon. If you just started to get Crohn's Disease symptoms, it's generally because of an imbalance of the microbial and not yet in a chronic state having a bigger influence on your immunity, becoming a full blown autoimmune disease. It is therefore much easier to treat at early stages of this condition then years down the road. If you have had your condition for many years and you have gone through most of the array of medical medications, your condition has probably flourished into a full blown autoimmune disorder because of the years of food sensitivities inflaming your body and medications, throwing your body completely off balance.

"The first wealth is health"

Ralf Waldo Emerson

3-Current medications for Crohn's Disease

These drugs are generally administered depending on where the disease is in the colon. They can be taken by mouth, enemas, or suppositories. There are other drugs that can be used to suppress the immune system. Crohn's Disease is defined as an autoimmune disease and for that reason, these drugs may be helpful. Some of these drugs have serious side effects so you should stay in contact with your medical doctor while taking them. Crohn's Disease patients also take iron supplements, antibiotics, and medicines to control diarrhea and pain relievers. Surgery removes both the colon and the rectum.

Anti-inflammatories

One of the first medications prescribed for mild to moderate Crohn's Disease is the drug Mesalamine (Liaida, Apriso, Canasa, Pentasa, and Asacol). These drugs usually work against bringing down inflammation in the colon.

Corticosteroids

Usually the first-line treatment drugs for Crohn's Disease are the corticosteroid drugs (budesonide Entocort, and Uceris). Steroids are often used locally through rectal infusion .

Immune System Suppressors

If you're diagnosed with Crohn's Disease and corticosteroids aren't helping your condition, your doctor may prescribe intravenous cyclosporine (Sandimmune) or infliximab (Remicade). These drugs are immunosuppressants, meaning they work by suppressing the activity of your immune system.

Biologics

Adalimumab (Humira) and Entyvio are the newest class of drugs available for treatment of Crohn's Disease. These drugs work via a monoclonal antibody that blocks an inflammation-causing protein.

Chances are you have been using one or more of these medications during your course of treatment with your gastrologist. Unfortunately, you have probably experienced the harmful side effects as well some are temporary and some could be permanent for the rest of your life. Some of these side effects include: joint pain, loss of eye sight, liver kidney damage, pain, bleeding, headaches, no energy, feeling week, nausea, bloating, and depression. And this is just to name a few. I could go on and on with their horrendous side effects. This is not the life that you want to live, suffering for the rest of your years and jumping from one med to another. You may even need to get on more meds now to manage the side effects of another med and so it turns into a vicious cycle and the only winners are the pharmaceutical companies.

What research is being done regarding Crohn's Disease? Research is ongoing to find other biological agents that are more helpful with fewer side effects in treating Crohn's. These may include: adalimumab, visilizumab, and alpha-4 integrin blockers. Research in Crohn's Disease is very active and many questions are still left to be answered. The cause of inflammation and best treatment options have yet to be defined. Researchers have recently identified genetic differences among patients. This information may allow them to select certain groups of people with Crohn's may react differently to different treatments.

You're reading this book for a reason and its probably isn't because you wanted to learn about these horrendous drugs with mega side effects. It's likely because you want to have your health back, a normal life back, and you don't want to take these traditional meds anymore. You may want to ween off these medications as soon as possible as you start having less and less symptoms of the disease and you should certainly do that, but it should be supervised by your doctor. I don't advocate that anyone drop their meds completely when you first start this program. Your meds will work as a bridge and of course give you some quality of life while you are getting better. Eventually you can start weening off the meds; you will feel and know when you can start weening of your meds as symptoms start disappearing or improving over time.

Caution you must contact your physician before easing off your medications and it should only happen under a physician's supervision

"The greatest wealth is health"

Virgil

4-How do we get Crohn's Disease?

The medical community really seems to have no clue as to how this condition starts in the body and for what reason. However, they do seem to have some belief that it has to do with both an autoimmune and intestinal microbial disorder. As many studies as they pursue, they seem to keep not analyzing peoples lifestyles and diet and previous antibiotic use. Over many years of study, I have come to the following conclusions of how Crohn's Disease starts in the body. I am sure that you probably fall into one of these categories as I did as well.

Let's start with your current or past lifestyle. Do you work at a very stressful job to the point where you find the stress effecting your nervous system to the point that you lose your appetite? The brain and your intestinal track are highly connected. Are you not eating much and drinking lots of coffee to keep you going? Or maybe you had a very dramatic situation in your life lately a death in the family, loss of a job, or major financial burdens or even a pregnancy.

You've been eating a terrible diet for many years, you eat out a lot at fast food restaurants, you eat a lot of processed foods, you snack on junk food on a regular basis, you've been drinking tons of pop and not enough clean water, or live foods such as fruits and veggies and clean healthy well balanced home cooked meals , you been eating a diet high in refined sugar. You have had your doctor prescribe antibiotics many times in your life and have used antibiotics through your various aliments in your life and your intestines have never felt well since then, maybe you experience bloating and indigestion on regular basis.

The combination of eating poor, unhealthy, processed, foods, combined with a very dramatic life event, added with stress and extended usage of antibiotics, this is what has lead your colon to go from a minor inflamed state to full blown condition like Crohn's Disease. You cannot expect your intestines to act like a trash can, put in nothing but garbage and expect not to get sick. Think back and also look at the correlation of when you got your Crohn's Disease and when your last antibiotic usage was. One seven day run of antibiotics is enough to destroy all the good bacterium in your intestines for close to 6 months. It's funny though, how the medical community does many studies, but they fail to do the most obvious studies that involve the most important factor as to lifestyle and what we put in our intestines.

5-My Personal Story with Crohn's Disease

You made it this far in the book, great! Now let me tell you my journey with this disastrous condition. I am sure all of you reading this book will be able to relate to some if not all of what I been through in my journey with Crohn's Disease. I will give you a little history about myself just before I was diagnosed with Crohn's Disease.

At the age of 18 I became infatuated with lifting weights and becoming a bodybuilder. I would think about it day and night; my whole life was bodybuilding. I would spend 7 days a week in the gym eating a high protein meals 6 to 7 times a day. My goal was to get as big as I could possibly get. As a young kid, I was always skinny. When I started lifting I was 137lbs and five foot ten inches in height, all I wanted was to be a huge bodybuilder and nothing was going to stop me; I did what it took to get there. At 21 years of age, I had reached a body weight of 225 lbs. and I was competing at national level bodybuilding contests. I was doing well and winning first place in many of the contests. I was living my dream and life was wonderful.

At the age of 26 years old, I was still lifting and still competing when one night I got up in the middle of the night with an extremely painful cramp on my right side of my abdomen. I had never had any health issues in the past. As matter of fact, because of my health regime since I was 18: eating healthy, training every day, not drinking or smoking, I was always healthy and felt as strong as an ox. As a matter of fact, I would never get colds or anything. This was the first time I actually felt something that really scared me. I was living with my dad at the time, and he suggested I get over to the hospital as soon as possible. Upon arrival, they ran some blood work, poked around on my abdomen, and concluded that I was a healthy guy. They told me that it was probably nothing and sent me home that same night with some pain killers. They told me not to worry, that the pain would go away, and I would be fine.

The next day I was still in a tremendous amount of pain, but I managed to control the pain with the pain meds they had given me. In my head I knew this was not normal and something had to be wrong. I had never had constipation before and I would use the toilet very regular multiple times a day. Later that same evening at about 10 pm, all of a sudden I had the worst pain I believe a human can ever experience from my abdomen. It was so painful that I went into shock and fainted with amount of pain.

I was rushed to the hospital by ambulance and upon arrival in my state of unconscious shock, they quickly determined that I had a ruptured appendix and that I would need to be rushed into immediate surgery to save my life. After awakening from surgery, I remember thinking to myself what just happened to me here, and how horrible I felt, but being the positive thinking person I was I figured I would be out of the hospital in no time and I would be back to my normal life and gym in no time.

One week after my admission, the doctors had not let me eat anything since my surgery. They had made it clear that any food in my system could cause more complications with my condition. This was a major disappointment for me as I was always concerned with losing weight and muscle loss. At this point, my abdomen had swollen to the point of almost looking like I was pregnant, and doctors seemed to be very concerned. They were trying different antibiotics at very high doses to bring down the infection that had become septic. This was a very serious state to be in, this was a state that can cause total organ failure and a potentially mortal state.

At week two, nothing had changed. My condition had gotten worse, my septic infection had gotten worse, and my abdomen was still swollen like a balloon. After still being on very high doses of antibiotics and several tries with huge needles to remove puss out of my abdomen, nothing had improved. Doctors approached me and let me know that unfortunately, they had to perform surgery again to save my life. They needed to go in and remove as much infectious puss as they could to clean me out and then close me back up again.

After my second surgery, a week later, doctors were confident things were looking better and that the septic infection was under control and that I was making progress. I was actually feeling better and my spirits were up, even though at this point my weight was deteriorating day by day, I just wanted to get out of the hospital and start eating again and get off the very harsh antibiotics that they had me on 24 hours a day on a drip system. It was now 6 weeks in a hospital since my arrival recovering when after several CAT scans to determine my level of infection in my abdomen they discovered that they had twisted my colon when they did my second surgery and that they would need to go in for a third surgery to straighten my colon. When I was told this, I could not of heard more devastating news, knowing I had to go under the knife again and stay in the hospital longer, recovering and taking more antibiotics. The next morning I had no choice, we decided to go into surgery hopefully for the third and last time. After surgery doctors had told me all went well. I was recovering well and two weeks later I was discharged with another borage of antibiotics to take home with me to continue taking for another 6 weeks to control any remaining infection in my body. Here I was at home happy in one sense, but still bed ridden in pain slowly recovering having had my abdomen cut down the middle, from my lower rib cage down to my groin area. It took a while before I could actually feel some comfort doing anything physical or even walk. So it took a while, but day by day I was gaining some weight back and slowly being able to physically get back on track.

After several weeks at home, I decided that after eating clean my whole life that I needed to eat whatever I could to gain my weight as fast as possible. So for the first time in my life I started eating a lot of garbage, a lot of fast food including burgers, pizza, pop, and cookies. I was eating things that I would never touch before. (Keep in mind I was still taking antibiotics at fairly high dosages.)

*****Now if you been reading carefully and paying attention to my story this is where the correlation that I will speak about in later chapter in this book as to why and how this disease manifests itself in our bodies so stay tuned for these details ****

It was at week number three when I started noticing that I was having regular bouts of diarrhea. Every few days I would have very runny stools. It would last a day or two and things would go back to normal and then return to diarrhea again and so forth for about a week or so. At that point I really thought nothing of it, I just figured it was probably normal and that I would be fine. I probably figured it was the antibiotics I was taking or the junk food and that it was no big deal. Little did I know at the time! The third week came and it just seemed to get worse, my trips to the bathroom had increased to 6-8 times a day. Now my diarrhea would be constant and very foul smelling. I remember at this point thinking, "What is going on?" And I knew that this was no longer normal and that I needed to see a doctor. So I booked an appointment for later that same week. While waiting for my doctor's appointment with my family doctor, things started to get worse. My trips to the bathroom were getting more frequent, and I was now starting to see blood in my stools. With the water in toilet turning red, and the more times I went to bathroom, the more blood I would see. It escalated to the point where it scared me so much that I called my dad and told him what was going on and he rushed me over to emergency at the hospital.

I had gone to the hospital with the fear of the worst. Terrible thoughts were going through my head: Did I have cancer? Was I dying? Had my infection gotten worse? All these horrible thoughts were going through my mind. I had suffered enough and now this was happening all over again.

After the doctors at the hospital had done several blood tests and several other stool sample tests, they booked me for a colonoscopy. They had not yet concluded anything, so I had to stay in the hospital overnight hooked up to an IV tube to rehydrate my body, as I was totally dehydrated from the frequent bloody diarrhea . The next day I was wheeled off into the colonoscopy test, this was not the most pleasant experience having a tube stuck up your anus, but I was anxious to find out what was going on with my body. I had completed the test and wheeled back to my room when about an hour later the Gastrologist walked in stood by my bedside and gave me the news that we all wish we had never heard.

He said, "Mr. Sousa after analyzing your test and doing a biopsy on your colon tissue you have Ulcerative Colitis and some Crohn's Disease in your smaller intestine! Your colon is inflamed and ulcerated he said he would write me up a prescription for a steroid med and it should help the inflammation..."

Having no idea what this disease was and never having heard about this disease before in my life, I didn't think much of it. I didn't even ask him any questions; I was just happy to hear that I didn't have cancer or anything life threatening. At least at that moment, I had felt some relief and peace of mind. I took the prescription and figured I will be OK after taking this medication. I asked him when I would be released from hospital. He said probably immediately and that I would have a follow-up appointment with him in 4 weeks' time.

After being released from the hospital about an hour later, I stopped at the drug store and picked up my prescription of Asacol 800mg, a very strong anti-inflammatory designed to reduce inflammation in the colon. I started taking two pills three times a day as per doctor's orders. About four days later I started feeling a bit better. I was seeing less blood and my frequency and urgency seemed to be getting better. My spirits were picking up and it looked like this hell that I had been experiencing was coming to an end.

In the meantime, I was also doing some research and after looking online. I got a major reality check that this was a very serious life-threatening disease. The doctors claim that you are stuck with it for life and there is no real cure, at least according to traditional medicine. But three weeks had gone by and my symptoms had gotten a lot better. I was no longer going to the bathroom 20 times a day and the blood was greatly reduced. But I was mostly still having diarrhea when I passed stool. My appointment or follow up was now a few days away and I figured that I would let the gastrologist know what I was experiencing and maybe he could adjust my meds and it would fix the diarrhea issue I was still having. Or maybe I could have a discussion with him about food and he could help me out. Oh, boy was I ever wrong!

Anyway, my appointment day came in anticipation that he would have a final fix for me. I rushed over there and even arrived early for my appointment. Now being much better informed, I had many questions for him and I needed answers. I remember this day like it happened yesterday. I walked in sat down in a chair across from his desk, he looked at me and said, "How is the Asacol working out for you?" I replied, "I feel better, the bathroom trips are much less, and blood loss has been better but still have diarrhea." To my dismay and shock! he looked at me and said, "My friend, you will have this disease for the rest of your life! And with these meds, they will only help you maintain some quality of life, but your colon will never function like a normal colon again." I remember sitting there for at least 45 seconds speechless in total shock. It was like I just heard a death sentence with almost tears coming to my eyes and trying to gain some sort of composer again. I remember looking up to him in total dismay and the first thing I got out of my mouth was, "But doctor, what if I change my diet?" He muttered back "Diet has nothing to do with this disease and it will not change anything. You can eat anything you want, but I would stay away from alcohol." In my head, I was thinking did I just hear that? Did he just say that? How can that be possible? Anyway, my appointment concluded with him increasing my dosage of Asacol and me leaving with a feeling of sadness and thinking how my future and life would be from this day on. I am sure many of you heard the same thing from your doctors, as this seems to be common protocol and you can likely relate to this feeling of being left helpless seeing your future in total hell with these words of complete disappointment from your doctors.

Driving home I remember so clearly like night and day how idiotic his statement of diet and food having nothing to do with this disease, in my head this just made no sense at all how can ulcers in my colon have nothing to do with food that was just ludicrous and made no sense what so ever, I mean I am not a doctor I had no medical degree but it's just plain common sense how can the doctor tell me such a thing.

I knew there was no way that this could be possible and I think right at that very moment is when I decided to take my health into my own hands and get all the facts and try and figure out this disease from every single aspect I was not going to leave my life and health in the hands of my gastrologist.

From that day on, I was obsessed with figuring this thing out. I would spend hours every day stuck to my computer reading countless medical articles, studies, and discussions on all the online Crohn's Disease and Crohn's forums. I spent hundreds of hours reading books and obsessively doing research. I knew I was going to figure this condition out or at least find things that could help me and others in the same boat. (Hence why I decided to write this book to help others as well as reach as many people as possible with my experiences and knowledge on the subject.)

For the next two years, I tried everything. I went through the full array of medications through my gastrologist. We tried them all with little to no success. Even if the condition had gotten a bit better for short time or at least my symptoms had gotten better, within a short period of time I was always back to the same flare ups and going through hell. I changed things in my diet and I tried every supplement out there. I even tried fecal infusions, which for some people they do have great success with, but for me it didn't work. I bought all sorts of shady supplements from India and China that claimed they were miraculous and cured Crohn's Disease, all with no avail and no success. It took me a long time to start figuring out what was actually working and what was not working before things started to change for me. I remember I was trying to ween off prednisone and I was experimenting with my diet different things: grain free, gluten free, low protein, and vegan, with some positive progress but not the meaningful results I wanted. At that time, I was reading Elaine Gotschalls book called "Breaking the Viscous Cycle." The book is all about the SCD Diet and it struck me like a bolt of lightning. The more I read, the more intrigued I was with the science behind it. It made total sense. Now here was a diet completely designed to help Crohn's Disease and Ulcerative Colitis patients. The next day I went out and purchased some of the food items that I needed and started following the diet. Things started to change after a few weeks and I started to feel better every day. I no longer was bloated. I was feeling better overall and for the first time I had some meaningful change for the better. I had found the right diet, now all I needed to do was find the raw compounds and supplements to help my body accelerate the healing progress. My journey continued. My research didn't stop and I tried tons of supplements until I came across the rights ones outlined in this book that brought me to a state of being completely symptom free. With these supplements and herbs I was making progress every day. I remember having tears of happiness in my eyes and thanking my Creator. Just from going to the bathroom and seeing normal stools. I was getting stronger and gained back the 52 pounds that I had lost. I was feeling energetic, loving life again, being social, spending more time with friends and loved ones, and finding love in my life again. I was also being able to get back into my biggest passion – the gym and lifting weights again.

I hadn't seen my doctor for about 5 months at this point and was feeling great! I was off all medications for well over 4 months. I had no reason to see him, but I had previously booked this appointment for a follow up, so I figured I would go see him either way. My appointment day arrived and on my way there I wasn't sure what I was going to say to him. After all, I had to tell him that I stopped taking his meds and that I was doing great, no symptoms what so ever and that I was back to normal. I decided I was just going to tell him straight up with no fillers. When I sat down in his chair he looked at me and said "You look like you gained some weight looks like we finally got your meds right." I looked at him and said, "No, I haven't been on any meds for over 5 months now." He looked at me in shock and asked "Why?" He then said, "Do you realize that you have to take these meds for rest of your life or this will come back tenfold as strong if you don't?" I looked at him and said, "Doctor I am completely symptom free. I am OK I am not sick anymore." He didn't say much for about 20 seconds I think he was in shock or upset. I am not sure what was going through his head, but he then said, "So you're not bleeding, no diarrhea, and you're only going to bathroom 1-2 twice a day?" I said "Yes!" I can tell that he was in disbelief and probably upset that I had not taken my meds. So he said, "Well let's get you scheduled in for a colonoscopy so we can see if there is still any inflamed tissue. You probably still have inflamed tissue in your colon." I take it by this comment that in his head it was impossible that I was symptom free without taking his prescription meds. Well it was true, regardless of his disbelief.

A week passed and it was my colonoscopy date. I wasn't looking forward to have them put that camera up my behind again, but at the same time I was feeling nervous about the results. What if the doctor was right? What if I still had inflamed tissue in my colon? That would mean I was still not healed! My test had gone well and I waited several days later for results from my family doctor. My family doctor had called me to come in for my results. In the back of my head I kept getting flash backs of what my gastrologist had told me – that my tissue was probably still inflamed even though I felt like a million bucks again. After sitting me down, my family doctor spit out the best words I had heard in my life in a long time. He said, "Your colon tissue shows no signs of any inflammation and all biopsies on tissue show completely healthy tissue with no sign of disease." This was music to my ears. That's when I knew then and there that the protocol that I was following was right, it had cured all my inflamed tissue in my colon. It was real, it was official, at this point I was onto something great and I had proven my protocol. Ten years later I am still enjoying life to the fullest with no signs of this disease. Our Creator has a plan for all of us and sometimes we have to suffer to come out of it better, stronger, and more knowledgeable. We all have a mission to fulfil and this was my mission, to help others so I decided to write this book and help as many people with this condition as I can. What took me years of research and knowledge you have it all in one book.

6-The Impact of Sleep & Stress on Your Body

In the balance of the following chapters until the end of this book, we will start looking at that parts of your 90-day program that will need to be implemented in your lifestyle. Every chapter in this book has an important impact on your results. We will start off by looking at the more obvious factors that have a direct impact on your condition and how you can change them.

Stress is known as one of the silent killers in the human body. Most people have no clue as to how bad leading a high stressful life leads to all sorts of diseases in the body. The medical community seems to at least understand that for Crohn's Disease patients stress stimulates new flare ups and has a direct correlation to worsening the condition. According to a recent study, being exposed to extreme stress causes a fivefold increase in the risk of a relapse of Crohn's Disease the next day. If you have Crohn's, this is not the time to be in a toxic relationship or experience financial problems. You must have the least amount of stress as possible if you want to heal your condition. Remove yourself from stressful situations and try and live stress free. Practice stress diminishing practices like deep breathing, meditation, and exercise for stress relief. You could also take up a hobby that keeps your mind happy and occupied and not thinking of the issues that cause you stress.

Sleep is a subject matter with us Crohn's Disease patients I hear about every day. It is usually patients complaining about not sleeping well or not getting enough of it because you're getting up all night to go to the bathroom. I like to say the bathroom was my new best friend at a point in my condition. Yes, it can be very hard on us, especially when we first get this condition and it's in a major state of flare up. Sleep is very hard to come by and the feeling of unrest dragging you down further, it does not help, and by any means does not make you feel cheery in the morning.

You will find this will only change with time over your 90-day period, as some of the symptoms of disease start to diminish. However there are some things that can help you until things get better. Just before you go to bed, take a very hot bath with Epson salts and maybe a few drops of eucalyptus oil in your bath water. These minerals naturally relax the body and help release sleep hormones. You can also get your doctor to give you a prescription for a sleeping drug, however these can be very addictive and assist with putting the body into an acidic state, so I don't recommend this route. Taking naps during the day also helps catch up on your missed sleep. You can also download sleeping music that helps relax the mind. There are several natural sleeping supplements that work very well. You can purchase these at your local health food store. The key is to get as much rest and sleep as you can. Sleep ensures the body's ability to heal and you need a lot of healing with this condition.

7-The liver and Gallbladder Detox Cleanse

Before we get into your 90-day program lets address one of the most important organs in your body, the liver! Why the liver you might ask? Well, the liver happens to be one of the most important organs in your body outside of looking at your brain and heart. The liver itself is responsible for over 400 different functions in the human body, and some of them go hand in hand with your gallbladder. So if we don't maximize the liver and gallbladder function, and bring them to a healthy state to where they can function as they were intended to, don't expect to heal your intestines. If these two organs are full of toxins and in simple terms just congested up, you're not going to heal, period!

Let me explain the correlation between healthy liver function, and the impact it has on treating Crohn's and Ulcerative Colitis. The liver's primary function is to detoxify the body neutralizing these chemicals and eliminating toxins out of the body, now if your liver is not functioning properly and is all congested then those toxins start spilling back into your intestines causing disease, and usually by that point you already have a chronic disease. I am sure you have heard of gallbladder stones, well the liver can also contain a massive amount of stones and liver globules as well. Your liver and gallbladder over time starts accumulating these stones, completely congesting both organs and not allowing them to function in the correct way supporting your digestion. Putting in a very simply in a manner that you understand... The liver produces all the right bile's and other substances that not only help with digestions but also helps neutralize intestinal acids, when this is not happening because of congestion these acids are so strong that they start eroding and causing inflammation in your intestines combine that with other factors like a terrible diet, antibiotic usage and you just created a chronic disease in your body .This is so important for detoxification. Your liver and gallbladder are so essential to proper digestion and the start of intestinal diseases so you must address this before we get into any part of this program. Make no mistake this has to be done, it cannot be skipped, it is a must and essential to healing your Crohn's Disease and Colitis. Not doing this would be like replacing the engine in your car with a new engine and then forgetting to put oil in the motor before you drive off. Let's address one of the most contributing factors to this disease and how it starts manifesting itself in your body.

Cleaning the liver with oils goes back thousands of years so this is nothing new even though you will not hear it from your traditional doctor they generally wait till the gallbladder is totally clogged with stones and opt to cut it out, or your liver is about to give out, and you get put on a liver transplant list. The bottom line is if you have a clean internal body you will not get diseases. When your pipes at home get clogged you call the plumber to clean them out will your pipes in your liver and gallbladder need to be clean as well for proper function.

Thanks to Dr Group, below you will find his 6-day Liver and Gallbladder cleanse his entire plan with a very particular diet to follow and the exact things and supplements you need to use to assist you in your cleanse. The instructions are laid out exactly as he has designed they have not been altered he has also addressed any common questions you may have regarding this cleanse. Keep in mind this is not the diet that we will be covering later in this book, this is only part of this 6-day cleanse diet and only to be used for this part of your program.

Dr Group's 6 Day Liver Cleanse Instructions

Supplies Needed for the Liver Cleanse

- The Liver Detox Kit (one bottle Liver Shield, one bottle Oxy-Powder)

- 1 (16 ounces) bottle of (Organic) Apple Cider Vinegar (ACV)

- 3 gallons of distilled or filtered drinking water

- 1 tablespoon of USP Epsom Salts

- 8 oz. of High-quality Cold Pressed Extra Virgin Olive Oil

- The recommended (organic fruits, vegetables (organic if possible)for the diet as listed below:

Following the diet program will give you great results but if for some reason if you feel that you're unable to follow this specific diet, at least try to limit your meat consumption to one portion every other day for lunch. Try eating fish and chicken, avoid red meat, as much as possible and incorporate healthier choices.

Ingredients for Days 1-4

Breakfast:	Lunch & Dinner:	Snacks:
Choose one of the following liver Detoxing fruits to eat or juice as much as you wish:	Use the following liver detoxing vegetables to make vegetable soup, juice, or salads:	In between your meals, you can eat a handful proportion of the below raw nuts and seeds:

• Watermelon	• Artichoke	• Sunflower seeds
• Papaya	• Asparagus	• Pumpkin seeds
• Kiwi	• Avocado	• Walnuts
• Plums	• Carrots	• Brazil nuts
• Pears	• Beets	• Almonds
• Apples	• Broccoli	
• Cherries	• Cabbage (green, purple or both)	
• Figs	• Kale	
• Grapefruit	• Brussel Sprouts	
	• Garlic	
	• Spinach	
	• Romaine lettuce	
	• Salad greens	
	• Onions	
	• Cauliflower	

Ingredients for Day 5 - Flush Day

Breakfast	Here is a list of the following liver cleansing fruits to eat or juice that you will be choosing from
	Papaya Watermelon Plums Kiwi Apples Pears Figs Cherries Grapefruit

Lunch	**Option #1 - Liver Detoxing Soup**	**Option #2 - Carrot Juice/Beet**
	1 Beet	3 Carrots
	2 Carrots	1 Beet
	1 Broccoli	2 Red Apples
	10 Garlic Cloves	6 Kale Leaves
	½ Onion	½ Lemon

	¼ Lemon 2 Bay Leaves 1 Teaspoon Himalayan Crystal Salt ½ Teaspoon Turmeric ½ Teaspoon Oregano	½ inch Ginger Root **Option #3** Water/ACV Mixture
Mid Afternoon	**snack Option #1**	**Option #2**
	Avocados Lime or Lemon Himalayan Crystal Salt	6-8 ounces of raw walnuts
		Option #3
		Mixture Water/ACV

Dietary Recommendations during Your Liver Detox

To get the most out of this liver cleanse, it's crucially important to follow a healthy diet to support your liver and colon cleanse. Try to incorporate as much of following dietary guidelines including eating organic to reduce any toxin exposure while cleansing your Liver.

- Try as much as possible to purchase organic or locally farm grown foods, conventional foods tend to be over-processed, and generally sprayed with harmful pesticides.

- Try to use only healthy oils in your diets such as flax seed, olive oil and hemp oils.

- Avoid dairy, cow's milk and cheese; instead try hemp or almond milk instead.

- Avoid any foods that may contain gluten, such as wheat, barley, cereals, white flour, pasta, bread, couscous, corn tortillas, crackers, pastries, cookies, chips, imitation fish products, fast food, hot dogs, and any fried foods.

- Avoid alcoholic drinks at all costs.

- Avoid diet pop and other products that contain any form of artificial sweeteners these can be, aspartame, acesulfame potassium, neotame, saccharin, and sucralose. Replace these with all natural sweeteners such as stevia, or honey.

- Avoid all foods that have high fructose corn syrup ingredients like molasses, corn syrup, sorbitol, dextrose, processed fructose, sucrose and of course white sugar.

- Replace the unhealthy table salt (sodium chloride) with the healthy Himalayan salt.

- Try to avoid any products containing soy. All soy contains pesticides and is genetically highly modified. The soybeans are also high in a type phytic acid which is extremely damaging to the intestinal tract.

- Caffeine used in moderation is acceptable however during your cleanse try consuming organic tea instead without creamers and try using natural sweeteners like raw honey.

What You should Expect During Your Liver Detox

Oxy-Powder may cause you to have watery stools, so make you are close to a bathroom. If your find your stools are liquid, this is not actually diarrhea but in actuality is a result of turning compacted feces in the digestive tract into a liquid and sometimes gas. Some people may experience what is commonly known as a healing crisis. This means that you may possibly feel worse during your liver cleanse than you did before you started the detox cleanse. This happens because of the accumulation of toxins in your system. These materials must be processed to be eliminated from the body. Don't get discouraged!

Before Starting: Prepare The Liver Cleanse Formula

The evening before you start your Liver cleanse, make the following 2-gallon formula and try to get a good night's rest.

How to instructions to Make the Liver Shield Cleanse Formula

- **Gallon #1:** Liver Shield Formula: Pour out 3 ounces from your 1st gallon of purified/filtered water and then add all of the Liver Shield formula pour entire contents in, and then add two heaping tablespoons of Apple Cider Vinegar (ACV). Shake few times and refrigerate.

- **Gallon #2:** Apple Cider Vinegar Mixture (ACV): Pour out 2 ounces from your 2nd gallon of filtered/purified drinking water and add 1 ounce of the same Raw Apple Cider Vinegar. Shake few times and refrigerate.

Day 1 - Start Your Liver Detox Cleanse

- **8:00am:** When you get up Eat a healthy Breakfast (look at breakfast diet options from day 1-4). Do not mix the fruits together!

- **9:00am:** Drink 8-ounces (gallon #1) of Liver Shield Cleanse Formula.

- **10:00-11:00am:** Water or a Snack (optional). Drink 12 ounces (gallon #2) of the Water/ACV Mixture.

- **12:00pm:** Drink 8-ounces (gallon #1)glass of the Liver Shield Cleanse Formula.

- **1:00pm:** Eat a healthy Lunch (look at lunch diet options from day 1-4). Drink only the Water/ACV Mixture (gallon #2) with your lunch.

- **3:00pm:** Drink 8-ounces glass of the Liver Shield Cleanse Formula (gallon #1).

- **4:00-5:00pm:** Water or a Snack (optional). Drink (gallon #2) 12 ounces of your Water/ACV Mixture.

- **6:00pm:** Drink one 8-ounce glass of the Liver Shield Cleanse Formula (gallon #1).

- **7:00pm:** Eat a Healthy Dinner Meal (look at dinner diet options from day 1-4). Drink only the Water/ACV Mixture (gallon #2) with your dinner meal.

- **8:00-10:00pm:** Before you go to sleep, take 4 capsules of Oxy-Powder. Try not go to bed very late, nothing past 10pm!

Day Two, Three, and Four of Your Liver Detox

You will need to follow the same instructions as Day 1, with a slight change, this time from **8:00-10:00pm:** Consume 6 capsules of the Oxy-Powder.

Day 5 of the Liver Cleanse – (Flush Day)🗓

8:00am to 10:00am – Breakfast (look at breakfast diet options for day 5). Do not mix your fruits! We highly recommend using watermelon on this day due to its high glutathione content.

After breakfast, you can now start prepping your Liver Cleanse Soup for lunch (the recipe is outlined below) if you choose Option #1. Drink the Water/ACV Mixture (gallon #2) as needed until lunch.

12:00pm – Your Lunch should be a Liver supporting meal. You have a choice from one of the listed three options for your lunch below:

Option #1 - Liver Cleansing Soup (Recommended)

To maximize the ability of the Liver to detox and cleanse, try to choose only the type of vegetables which are high in Sulphur and Glutathione. Sulphur helps the liver cleanse out of the body harmful chemicals.

The following ingredients are included in the liver cleanse soup (Soup Option #1)

- 1 Beet (Chopped)

- 2 Carrots (Chopped)

- 1 Cup Broccoli (Chopped)

- 10 Garlic Cloves (Minced)

- ½ Onion (Chopped)

- ¼ Lemon

- 2 Bay Leaves

- 1 Teaspoon Himalayan Crystal Salt

- ½ Teaspoon Turmeric

- ½ Teaspoon Oregano

- There are other liver cleansing foods you can use: asparagus, kale, artichoke cabbage, cauliflower and brussel sprouts can also be added to the soup.

To prepare the Liver Cleanse Soup:

Wash all your vegetables well. Finely chop ingredients. Pour about 32 ounces give or take of filtered/distilled water into a large soup pot. Add all of the prepared ingredients to the water. Bring the soup up to a boil, then reduce the heat, and simmer on low heat temperature for at least one hour. You can now eat this soup for lunch. After your meal, refrigerate the remaining balance of your soup for so you can eat it for tomorrow's lunch (Day 6).

Option #2 - Beet/Carrot Juice (Soup Option #2):

- Peel and juice all the ingredients in a blender until soupy consistency is achieved.

- 3 Carrots (peeled)

- 1 Beet (peeled)

- 2 Red Apples (cut)

- 6 Kale Leaves

- ½ Lemon (peeled)

- ½ inch Ginger Root

Option 3: Your (Water/ACV Mixture) - If you do not feel hungry and if you think that you can fast through lunch, then drink several 8-ounce glasses of the Water/ACV Mixture (gallon #2) as you can.

2:00pm - Mid-Afternoon Small Snack. This will now be your last meal that you will be eating for the day. Choose only one of the following options:

Option #1: Avocados, Lime or Lemon, & Himalayan Crystal Salt. Eat 2-3 avocados. Season with Himalayan salt and some fresh lime/lemon juice to taste. Avocados assist the body in producing glutathione, which is required for the liver to cleanse harmful toxins out.

Option #2: Eat 6-7 ounces of uncooked raw organic walnuts. Walnuts contain large amounts of the amino acid arginine, and this is necessary to help the liver detoxify ammonia. Make sure you chew walnuts thoroughly until they are fully liquefied before swallowing.

Option #3: Water Meal. If you are not feeling any hunger and you can fast through the afternoon, drink as much of the Water/ACV Mixture (gallon #2) as you can.

7:00pm – (USP) Epsom Salt: Mix 1 full tablespoon of Epsom Salt in 8 ounces of warm filtered/purified water. Try and drink it as fast as you can. It's not the most pleasant taste; It is also advisable to be near a bathroom some individuals may experience liquid stools within a short time 20-30 minutes after ingesting.

8:30pm to 9:00pm: Drink the Extra Virgin Olive Oil & Juice: Drink ¾ cup (6 ounces) of extra virgin, cold pressed olive oil. You can add a small amount (approximately .2 tablespoons) of freshly squeezed, grapefruit, or lemon juice. This can be added to improve the oils taste.

How Should you Drink the Olive Oil: It's imperative to drink all 6 ounces of the oil; below are three approaches if you're having a hard time drinking the oil:

Approach #1: Refrigeration will thicken the oil if you place it in the fridge for a few hours before ingestion, this will make it go down quickly.

Approach #2: You can also thin the oil by placing the oil in a jar and then mixing ½ cup of fresh Lemon/grapefruit into the oil and shaking until it thins out.

Approach #3: To reduce the oil taste and texture, gather two cups, straw, and some of the juice. Place the juice in one cup, olive oil in the other, and use the straw to alternate sipping between the two cups.

Now, this is very critical, immediately after ingesting the oil, go to your bed and lie only on your right side, try tucking your knees up to your stomach for at least 30 minutes.

After laying on your right side for 30 minutes, you can now stretch out and go to sleep on any side you wish. If you experience any form of cramping, walk around for few minutes or so and then head back to bed. You may also feel some nausea during the night. This is mostly due to the release of all your Liver and Gallbladder stored toxins. This is entirely normal, and a great sign that the liver cleanse is working as it should.

If you get the feeling and your wanting to vomit, do so, as this will help eliminate toxins. Do not take any Oxy-Powder on this evening.

Congratulations! You have just finished your first liver cleanse!

What Should you Expect After the Liver Cleanse

When waking in the morning, you must immediately take six capsules of Oxy-Powder. This will assist your intestinal tract and help the body flush the stones out that have been released from the liver and gallbladder while you were sleeping at night. Now, for breakfast, only eat fruit. For lunch, you can eat the leftover portion of the liver cleanse soup. Have a healthy dinner such as a light salad with some protein.

If you want to see what the stones look like, they should appear when you have a bowel movement for one to two days. You can use a cheap colander placed over the toilet to collect any stones and then rinse away the fecal matter in the sink. You will be shocked at what actually comes out of you.

If you still feel that you are experiencing indications after doing your third flush, this probably a sign you will require additional cleanses. The most we have I have heard of someone completing is 20 back-to-back Liver cleanses before their indications were reduced.

Frequently Asked Questions:

1) Can this liver cleanse be done if the gallbladder has been removed?

Yes! When the gallbladder has been surgically removed, the wondrous human body generally compensates in one shape or another for its absence. The bile duct that is found on the visceral side of your

Liver will increase in size to compensate over for the task of storing bile. Some post-surgery patients experience diarrhea, including Irritable Bowel Syndrome whereas others have no post-surgery symptoms whatsoever.

Keeping the Liver clean, is essential as it no longer has it's supporting organ called the Gallbladder, so it is vital to the ones who have had gallbladder surgery promote a healthy and vigorous digestive system.

2) Sea Salt vs. Epsom. Which salt is better to use?

Epsom Salts are mandatory for the liver flush. They not only provide a very strong laxative action in the colon, but the Magnesium Sulphate relaxes the bile ducts, there making it easier to pass larger stones. The taste of Epsom salts is quite unpleasant, to say the least, but regardless of taste, it is an essential ingredient when performing a liver flush. Sea Salt such as Himalayan will not have the same effect; unfortunately, there are no alternatives or substitutes.

3) How do you know if your liver is clean?

Everyone's results will differ depending on lifestyle, diet, exercise, and age as well as their physical and emotional stress levels. The liver and gallbladder are truly never 100% clean since if you study their intended function is to metabolize toxic material. In terms of generally speaking, most people usually require about three cleansing sessions followed by several periodic cleanses few times per year for maintaining your liver. One of the best ways is to judge from the lessening of your indications. Many of these indications will simply just resolve after the several cleanses. While others individuals may take 6 or 7 consecutive, cleanses and others even require the identification and solutions for other factors, i.e. supplementation, environmental, emotional trauma, and nerve damage. The stools may continue to be runny or very loose due to the oxidation process from using Oxy-Powder. If you notice a foul smell in the initial stages of cleansing, this is normal. Over time, you will notice a decrease in foul-smelling bowel movements. Normal and healthy bowel movements usually are extracted out of the body in a very timely manner, with the healthy stool usually being lighter brown in colour, relatively smooth, in appearance.

4) Will I go through a healing crisis?

Yes, it's a good possibility that you may experience a healing crisis. This is a phenomenon that sometimes occurs during detoxification and cleansing of the body and liver. It's a real possibility that you may feel worse during and after your cleanse than you did before you got started it. The accumulation of toxic material in your liver after so many years must be processed to be eliminated from the body. This process can cause certain physical indications by these toxins as they are further metabolized in the body. The most common indications are usually: headaches, fatigue, minor skin rashes, lack of mental clarity, muscle or joint ache, irritability, mood swings, and difficulty sleeping. Some people can experience multiple indications at once while others have one or none at all. These indications will go always disappear in 2 to 3 days as the body naturally rids itself these toxins. However, many people report feeling fabulous and full of energy and with an increased sense of well-being after the initial liver cleanse. If after your cleanse you feel worse, I strongly suggest that you should continue with the cleansing process and at least perform a few more cleanses. In addition, also lifestyle changes adopting an organic, non-processed food diet and drinking only filtered/purified water with raw apple cider vinegar and of course with plenty of rest may help you to feel better. Massage and heat saunas may also contribute to eliminating toxins from the body.

5) Can I take any Medications while I am performing a Liver Cleanse?

It is always suggested before you proceed with anything, consult with your personal doctor regarding any prescription medications that you may be taking while performing a liver cleanse. However be sure to only take your prescription meds well away from the Liver formula and also to take your Oxy-Powder 3-6 hours apart from your meds.

8-Diet in Relation to Crohn's Disease

You have now reached the chapter where I will teach you exactly what you need to do in the next 90-days to treat your Crohn's Disease.

Do you ever hear that saying that you are what you eat? Well, that has to be the most truthful statement you have ever heard. Our health is fully determined by what we eat, the water we drink, and other environmental influences on or bodies. You can't fuel your body with junk food or very poor quality food and expect to have great health.

Let's start your healing journey by fixing the most basic element, the food that we put in our mouths that promote a healthy healing environment, and provide your body with all the basic healing elements, foods and herbs that are rich in all the essential minerals and vitamins, proteins and other healing factors. This will bring your body to self-heal itself from a chronic ailment like Crohn's Disease.

I cannot put a greater emphasis on this chapter as the most important part that you need to change if you want to cure your condition. This is the most basic and most important part. This is a must do in your healing journey! If you do not change your eating habits, you will not see the results, so please follow this as much as you possibly can. Have you ever heard this saying? A wise man built his house on a rock foundation, but the foolish man built his house on a sand foundation.

If you have Crohn's Disease, you have some sort of food sensitivity. Now what does a food sensitivity mean? It means that you have some sort of inflammatory reaction to a particular food or what's contained in the food. For example, gluten is present in wheat products so when you eat a slice of wheat bread you will get an inflammatory reaction in the body. These inflammatory reactions as explained in previous chapters eventually lead to a leaky gut and that eventually leads to a chronic illness like Crohn's Disease, and there for causing an autoimmune condition in your body.

So what do we do? I suggest if you can afford it, go get an IGG test to determine what foods that you have a sensitivity to. There are many labs all over the U.S., Canada, and Europe that provide these IGG FOOD SENSITIVITY tests, or you can contact your local natural practitioner clinic and see if it's available through them. These tests usually range from several hundred to about five hundred dollars. This is highly suggested so that you can eliminate these foods immediately from your diet so you are not contributing to the inflammatory state or causing any further inflammation in the body and colon. This is extremely important. Do some research online and you will find lots of information on where you can get IGG test done in your local area.

OK now let's look at what you can actually eat and what diet you should follow to start changing the bacterial state of your colon and reduce the inflammation that is causing the autoimmune condition.

Along with the elimination of foods with your IGG test, this diet below is a must! Again you will not see results if you do not follow this diet.

SCD diet: Specific carbohydrate diet. Hundreds of thousands have had success with this diet. And you will also find that this alone will change your condition for the better within a reasonable time period of 90 days. The allowed carbohydrates are monosaccharides and have a single molecule structure that allows them to be easily absorbed by the intestine wall. Complex carbohydrates are not allowed. Complex carbohydrates that are hard to digest can feed harmful bacteria in our intestines. This can also cause them to overgrow producing by-products and inflaming the intestine wall. The specialized diet works by starving out these bacteria and restoring the balance of bacteria in our gut. The SCD diet also reduces inflammation by eliminating foods that contribute to inflammation, all these Gluten containing starches and grains are all eliminated on this diet promoting a healthy colon with much less inflammation.

The Specific Carbohydrate Diet™ is biologically correct because it is species appropriate. The diet we evolved to eat over millions of years was predominantly one of meat, fish, eggs, vegetables, nuts, and low-sugar fruits. Our modern diet which includes starches, grains, pasta, legumes, and bread has only been consumed for a

10,000 years. In the last hundred years, the increase in complex sugars and chemical additives in the diet has led to an increase in health problems ranging from bowel disorders to obesity and brain function disorders. We have not successfully adapted to eat this modern diet. It, therefore, makes sense to eat the diet we evolved with.

The Specific Carbohydrate Diet™ was clinically tested for over 50 years by Dr. Haas and biochemist Elaine Gottschall.

The following online link http://www.breakingtheviciouscycle.info/legal/listing/ provides a list of foods that are allowed (legal) and foods that are not allowed (illegal) while following the Specific Carbohydrate Diet.

If you can afford to only use organic vegetables, fruits, and hormonal free grass feed animal meat only, it is highly advised and will only speed up your healing big time. If you can't do the SCD diet because it's too strict, at the very least follow a dairy free, wheat free, sugar free, and most important a gluten free diet. This is a must!

9-Curring Your Crohn's Disease in 90 Days

Beyond outlining my personal story and stressing the great importance of following the SCD Diet as the most essential component of your 90-day program, in this chapter you will get to read about your 90-day program. You'll learn what supplements to take, how to take them, where to get them, and how you should eat. Let's look at the details, starting with supplementation and herbs.

Supplements and herbs

As we now look at the building blocks, what I call supplements and herbs to provide your body with the right minerals and healing compounds that will may balance what is currently lacking. An example such as you might be deficient in vitamin D or B complex. Another example is iron, which is usually the case with Crohn's Disease patients; they tend to be anemic due to the blood loss, a very low deficiency of iron. We will also be looking at some miraculous compounds that will help you ween off your current meds such as the biologics, immunomodulators, steroids and harsh anti-inflammatory meds that we all take for this disease and unfortunately they all carry horrendous side effects.

Cannabis oil: First and foremost, let's look at the most important supplement you can take. Cannabis has to be the most effective supplement that will change your condition with a noticeable difference in a week's time or less. As is true with many disorders, cannabis has been used for centuries to treat the symptoms of Crohn's Disease. The reason that cannabis is an effective treatment for these disorders is that cannabis can significantly limit intestinal inflammation. According to a statement issued by The Crohn's Disease Foundation of America in 2012, compounds found in the marijuana plant closely mimic endocannabinoids (molecules that occur naturally in the body) and have been shown to play an important part in decreasing gastrointestinal inflammation. Studies have also shown that Cannabis also works inside the body the same way that prednisone does the popular Crohn's Disease medication without the horrendous side effects.

Many people benefit from the anti-inflammatory properties of medical cannabis. IBD patients have been shown to have more cannabinoid receptors in the tissue of the colon than people without IBD. This means that people affected by Crohn's Disease are likely to respond to the anti-inflammatory properties of medical marijuana.

Researchers at the Institute of Gastroenterology and Liver Diseases at Chaim Sheba Medical Center have discovered that medical cannabis can help improve the quality of life in people affected by Crohn's Disease. This study also found that medical cannabis can stimulate the appetite in patients, resulting in healthy weight gain and an overall improvement in symptoms.

The same study found that after 3 months of treatment with medical marijuana, patients affected by Crohn's Disease enjoyed a better quality of life and a drastic decrease in pain reduction. These results were reported without accompanying side effects.

Researchers at the Sire Manchester Hospital in England published a study that found that IBS patients who used medical cannabis reported improved diarrhea symptoms and a decrease in pain.

While it is clear that cannabis is a valuable treatment option for patients with Crohn's Disease, researchers have found that there is a specific strain combination with cannabis oil that is ideal. You can smoke it, but some case studies have suggested that the oil is much more effective for Crohn's Disease patients. Studies have shown that a hybrid combination and THC and CBD content is key, with as close as the possible ratio of 50/50 percent of THC to CBD ratio oil has been most effective for me and others that have used this protocol. What I have done was buy two oils, one high in CBD and one high in THC and I have mixed them together to get the best ratio combination. I have yet to find a legal lab that produces a ratio that is fairly close. The recommended dose of cannabis oil should be approximately one gram per day total. For your first three weeks you should start with 0.3 ml to 3 times a day. First thing in the morning, on empty stomach, at some point mid-day, and your last dose should be administered just before you go to sleep. Use a typical insulin syringe to measure your dosage and spaced out evenly during waking hours. After your first few months at this dosage, you should increase your intake to about one gram and a half 1-1/2 grams to 1-3/4 grams total for one day administered approximately every 4 hours throughout the day.

As the law stands now, it is not legal for use or sale in many countries and states so make sure that you are complying with your country or state laws before using marijuana. Use it at your own risk, considering this there are dozens of high-quality studies that illustrate the fact that medical marijuana serves an important purpose in treating and alleviating the symptoms of painful IBD disorders. In addition to relieving pain, muscle cramps, anxiety, insomnia and inflammation, certain strains of cannabis also promote appetite, produce weight gain, and enhance the mood of affected patients.

*****I also suggest that patients should not try to drive their cars until they become more accustomed to the effects of the oil, after which they are then able to drive safely once more. Once you become used to the effects of the oil it does not impair your ability to drive in anyway, because unlike alcohol and many pharmaceuticals, this oil does not impair your motor skills***

You must also consult your physician to make sure the oil has not adverse effects if you have any other health conditions before starting cannabis use.

Colostrum is our first food early in life. We get it from our mother immediately after birth. It was designed by nature to defend and protect us from infection and help us grow healthy and strong. It has unsurpassed immune, autoimmune, allergy, gastrointestinal, athletic, diet and anti-aging performance. It is our first antibiotic and antiviral and has had more continued use than any other substance for health in cultures throughout the world than any other health product. It is studied more than any other nutritional substance around the world. Immunoglobulins from colostrum were used by Dr. Jonas Salk to develop the first oral polio vaccine. John Heinerman, Ph.D, one of the world's leading medical anthropologists and the author of more than fifty books on health and nutrition, stated that without colostrum's development by nature we would be extinct.

Looking at one of the nature's most effective and powerful foods. As our first food, it provides the infant with the ability to ward off and fight infection of all types and helps stimulate cellular growth in the colon. It stimulates cell growth in the intestines to close stomach and intestinal openings that are present in patients with Crohn's Disease and Crohn's disease and also helps build the mucosa wall in the colon. Colostrum's components reach all of the body structures to enhance growth and create perfect health. Colostrum readies the body for nutrition and helps populate the bowel with healthy flora and enhances their growth and colonization.

This incredible supplement can be bought on www.Amazon.com. Make sure you buy a high-quality colostrum; I only recommend Sovereign Laboratories and Immune Tree colostrum. I have done research on both these companies and they are the best in the industry as far as colostrum production. Both of these companies provide colostrum in the powder format and are manufactured the right way taken from grass fed cattle, harvested within the first 8 hours of a calf being born this process maintains the beneficial and integral parts of the colostrum.

So how do you take colostrum? I recommend you should start with buying a one-kilo container size of the powder format because you will be taking quite a bit of this supplement. The recommended doses for Crohn's Disease patients would be two taps. Three times a day, mixed with filtered water or bottled water. Again ideally you should take this with 10oz of water first thing in the morning on an empty stomach and wait at least 30 minutes before you eat anything followed by a mid-day dosage and again before you go to bed always 30 minutes before you eat on empty stomach.

Probiotics are another essential and extremely important product that needs to be consumed by Crohn's Disease patients as part of your healing journey. Probiotics hold the key not just for better health and a stronger immune system, specifically treating digestive issues. Probiotics are bacteria that line your digestive tract and support your body's ability to absorb nutrients and fight infection. Your body has ten times more probiotics in your gut than cells in your body. If you don't have enough probiotics, the side effects can include digestive disorders, skin issues, candida, autoimmune disease, and frequent colds and flu, and a major contributor to making your Crohn's Disease condition worsen until you get the bacterium in the digestive colon in balance.

Your gut contains both beneficial and harmful bacteria. Digestive experts agree that the balance of gut flora should be approximately 85 percent good bacteria and 15 percent bad bacteria. *Dysbiosis* is a condition when this ration gets out of balance. which means there's an imbalance of too much of a certain type of fungus, yeast or bacteria that negatively affects the body. By consuming certain types of probiotics foods and supplements, you can help bring these ratios back into balance. So how much probiotics should you consume on your 90-day journey? I believe that you should be consuming two forms for optimal results one format is in a food source, such as naturally fermented foods like *Kimchi, Miso, Non-pasteurized sauerkraut, Coconut kefir, Kombucha and homemade yoghurt* if you don't have a dairy food sensitivity. These should be consumed with every meal in small amounts; the second format is a capsule supplement. The reason for this is that you should introduce as many different diverse probiotic microbiomes strands as possible. Now when you purchase your probiotic supplement, please make sure that you only buy it if it's being stored in a refrigerator. However if it's sitting on a shelf outside of the fridge, do not buy these low-grade products. Probiotics are alive bacterium that needs to be kept in the refrigerator. Here are a few of the high quality brands that I suggest for consumption on your program. The following brands are recommended: *Natural Factors, Genestra Brands, Renew Life, Garden of Life, Axe Naturals and Jarrow Formulas.* Look for strains like *bacillus coagulants, saccharomyces bollard, bacillus subtitles, lactobacillus rhamnose,* and other cultures. The recommended usage for Crohn's Disease patients would be to take 3 capsules with your colostrum in the morning as this increase's the potency of the probiotic. Then 2 more capsules with every meal throughout the day. You should also purchase if possible a brand that has as many diverse stands in a bottle as possible the average stands available are usually between 8 and high as 30 always aim for the higher strand count if possible, this will give you a better variety of bacterium introduction to the thousands of healthy bacterium already in your colon. Research continues to prove that probiotics benefits and side effects go far beyond what we previously thought.

L-Glutamine is one of the most important nutrients for your intestine that benefits your health if you have any type of digestive issue, such as irritable bowel syndrome (IBS), an inflammatory bowel disease like Crohn's disease, Crohn's Disease, diverticulosis, diverticulitis, leaky gut or any of the issues associated with leaky gut. L-Glutamine is an amino acid that provides the mucosal cells of the intestine with the right energy source to heal damaged tissue or ulcerated tissue.

Why L-glutamine? Although it's an amino acid that is used frequently as a sports and fitness supplement, it has been found to modulate the immune system and protect the mucosal protective layer in the colon. Studies have demonstrated that L-glutamine improves blood flow to the damaged tissue in the intestine with patients that have Crohn's Disease. L-glutamine also is able to promote and reduce leakiness of the gut which may help reduce inflammation in the intestine. I have also found that it gives me instant relief at times with pain and very soothing feeling in your colon after drinking a glass of water at room temperature (very Important).

How do you take L-glutamine? It's good practice to take 20 grams with your other supplements first thing in the morning on an empty stomach with at least 10 Oz of water it can be mixed with colostrum and probiotics for great results. Followed by another 20 grams before you go to bed with 100oz of filtered or bottled water. This has to be one of the fastest acting supplements, most feel very soothing feeling after taking L-Glutamine. So 20 grams twice a day is your required dosage. You can purchase L-Glutamine almost at any fitness store or health food store in any country; it's a very readily available supplement.

Sodium Butyrate is another beneficial supplement as part of your 90-day program. Although several studies have shown the benefits of butyrate enemas in Crohn's Disease patients, In conclusion, there results also show that oral administration of sodium butyrate improves mucosa lesion and attenuates the inflammatory profile of intestinal mucosa, locally draining lymph nodes and Peyer's patches of DSSinduced UC. There results also highlight the potential use of butyrate supplements as adjuvant in UC /Crohn's treatment. How do you take it ? Your suggested use is two 600 mg capsules in-between meals on an empty stomach twice a daily. You can purchase this product on www.Amazon.com or your pick it up at your local health food store or online supplement suppliers.

Phosphatidyl Choline: Many studies show the hypothesis of an anti-inflammatory effect of phosphatidyl choline in Crohn's Disease. Examinations show retarded release oral phosphatidyl choline is effective in alleviating inflammatory activity caused by Crohn's Disease. This supplement has shown the ability to help and assist in combination with your other supplements to reduce inflammation bring better functionality reducing urgency in the colon. This supplement should be taken in the following manner 2 420mg capsules twice a day, one in the morning and once before bed. This supplement can be found relatively cheap and purchased at most health food stores or can also be ordered from www.Amazon.com.

Perm A vite: Made by a company called *Allergy Research Group* contains nutrients known to nutritionally support the lining of the gastrointestinal tract, such as Cellulose, MSM, Slippery Elm, N-Acetyl-D-Glucosamine, and Glandular Complex with Epithelial Growth factor. These compounds greatly help and accelerate the healing of the damaged tissue providing all the raw nutrients the body requires to repair these damaged tissues.

90 Essential Minerals & Vitamins:

True health and wellness is only possible if it radiates from a solid, fundamentally-sound center. There is a core group of 90 essential nutrients that have the most positive effect in bringing health to the human body's complex and multi-dimensional systems.

Did you know that only 8-12 percent of the nutritional supplements on the shelf are absorbed by your body? That means that approximately 90 percent of supplements are flushed down the drain. That's why I emphasize always buying high quality supplements.

The brand (Youngevity's) supplements are 90-98% absorbable! Why is there such a difference? The secret is there exclusive source of plant-derived minerals that dramatically increase bioavailability (absorbability). They produce a product called (Tangy Tangerine) which is their mineral and vitamin formula. In my opinion this is the best product on the market in this category. What I highly recommend you use on your 90 day program. The product comes with a 5 gram scoop; you should take one scoop a day with water.

Your body will require all these vitamins and minerals as part of the raw materials in the body used to heal your Crohn's Disease condition if your body is missing a mineral or several as they work in conjunction with each other so therefor you require all of them in your diet and program so the body can start the healing process.

Herbs: Why herbs? I like to call them alkalizing herbs, these herbs play a huge role in helping you heal your condition by helping the body into a better alkaline state which is ideal to heal any condition in the body , why Alkaline you ask? Well when we have been eating processed food, taking medications, drinking alcohol and eating high amounts of protein the body becomes very acidic and this is an environment that promotes disease and not good health. So therefore we must look at getting the body into a more acidic state buy consuming these alkalizing herbs, but also provide the body with blood cleaning properties, providing the body with useable iron, and helping reduction in inflammation and pain.

Sasapirilla (*Smilax, Hemidesmus indicus*) this herb has anti-inflammatory, antiulcer, antioxidant and very   high in iron properties.

Guaco (*Mikania Guaco, Mikania Glomerata, Leaf of Life*) this herb also has very high anti-inflammatory properties highly used for inflammation in the digestive tract and as an antibacterial for candida and yeast over growth in digestive tract.

Burdock Root (*Arctium Lappa*) is loaded with anti-inflammatory properties, blood cleansing, anti-fungus anti-viral and rich in iron as well.

The best way to take these herbs as they are not always readily available at your local food store in capsule format or available on www.amazon.com, is to buy the herb in bulk from this online store www.bulkherbstore.com or your local herbal store. The best way to approach this is to mix the 3 herbs in equal parts in a bag or bowl and then boil the leaves, roots and stems for at least 25 minutes and then let it sit for about 25 minutes before you drink it. This process is to insure that that all the essential properties are seeped into the tea that you will be drinking , you should then filter the tea through a fine strainer and drink the tea. The program suggests drinking at least one full liter of this combo tea everyday it will really slow down your inflammation and help with abdominal pain.

"The fruit thereof shall be for meat and the leaf thereof for medicine."

Bible Verse Ezekiel. 47:12,

Fiber: Mostly known as roughage, mostly from veggies and fruits etc., it's the indigestible part of live plant foods that travels through our digestive tract. Absorbing fluids along its movement in your colon and easing excretion of stool out of your body. So let's look at the importance of fiber in your 90-day program. By adding extra fiber to your diet later down the road with your 90 day journey is highly recommended let me explain! When you start your journey your colon is in a very inflamed state the mucosa is inflamed bleeding basically if you imagine a cut on your arm that's bleeding well that's what Crohn's Disease is, in your colon ulcerations small holes that bleed. When you first start your healing 90 day program you should only eat cooked fiber in other words your veggies should be cooked so the fiber is not so harsh on your mucosa wall ,acting as a sand paper and possibly causing more irritation and more bleeding ,it is helpful not to eat any significant amounts of raw veggies and some raw uncooked fruits at first, but as your colon is healing and the mucosa layer is sealing up and no longer bleeding you can slowly start adding raw veggies back in and supplemental fiber into your diet also. Flax seeds- ground up are your best source of supplemental fiber. You can add this in at your discretion as you feel your symptoms are no longer present specially bleeding and pain with formed stool for at least several months.

Juicing: The juice of fresh fruits and vegetables is the richest available food source of vitamins, minerals and enzymes. Usually, a person cannot consume enough raw fruits and vegetables in a day to nourish a starving body that is normally very much depleted in Crohn's and Colitis patients due to the condition of the intestines. This is a fact that was always true, but especially these days when the body requires these nutrients when we are bombarded with a major amount of environmental toxins. You probably don't have the time to sit there and eat 5 pounds of carrots but you can certainly drink that there equivalent in a delicious glass of carrot juice. If you haven't invested in buying a juicer yet then I suggest you go out and get one it will be the best investment in your health that you can make.

What should I juice for my Crohn's condition? Well, you should use bananas as a base. Bananas coat your intestines, help soothe the colon, they are full of magnesium, they promote relaxation of the muscles in the bowel walls, and really helps to heal the ulcerations. Cabbage is probably right up there with Bananas as far as being full of bioflavonoids. Some people have healed ulcers in their stomach just by drinking cabbage juice alone and nothing else. These two are probably the best fruit and veggie you can consume for this disease. You can add apples as they are wonderful at detoxing the colon, sure you have heard the saying "an apple a day keeps the doctor away". It is also very important to juice green leafy veggies like kale, parsley, beets and carrots very rich in Iron and folic acid which is essential for Crohn's patients to consume as they are always lacking in these important minerals that help wound healing in the intestines. These are also great sources of vitamin C needed for mucous membrane healing. If you add probiotics to your juices, especially to juices with bananas, the good probiotics flourish as they use bananas as a food source in your body.

Bone broth: made from beef bones, chicken, fish and lamb bones have all been staples in the traditional diets all over the world for thousands of years. Bone broths are very nutrient-dense. The bone stock was a way that our ancestors made use of all parts of animals that were consumed. Inedible bones and marrow, knuckles, and feet, tougher meats, tendons and even ligaments were boiled then simmered over for several days. Simmering causes the bones to release all the healing compounds like glutamine, proline, glycine, and collagen, these all have the incredible power to heal your gut.

The bone broths contain essential minerals in natural formats that your body can readily absorb: Sulphur, silicon, calcium, magnesium, phosphorus, and others. Broths also contain chondroitin and glucosamine, these are pricey supplements that are sold to heal joints and also reduce inflammation. Broths contain almost everything your body needs to repair your gut and your joints. Most people that suffer from Cohn's or Colitis also have joint problems since the body is taking calcium from your bones due to the inflammation in your gut which leads to joint issues. Stock and soup made with fish carcasses or fish heads provide iodine and thyroid-strengthening substances as well all these elements help with your Cohn's condition.

Benefits of Bone Broths: Bone broths are a very simple tasty liquid, but it is also filled with tremendous health benefits far beyond what you might think.

1. Heals a leaky gut. The beneficial gelatin in bones released into the broth protects and heals the mucosal lining of the intestinal tract. Amino acids such as l-glutamine in broth are the main amino acid your gut uses to repair the gut lining.

2. Broth helps Overcome most food intolerances and also allergies. By healing a leaky gut condition such as when you have Crohn's or Colitis you can resolve issues related to food sensitivities and allergies. Because these

sensitivities are caused by undigested large food particles seeping out of a leaky gut and into your bloodstream, triggering an immune response. Broth helps in preventing this issue.

3. Bone stocks help Heal joint pain and inflammation. The glucosamine in the stock stimulates the growth of new collagen, repairs damaged joints, reduces pain and inflammation in the colon.

4. Broth Facilitates new bone formation and repair. Minerals, such as magnesium and phosphorus found in bone broth repairs our bones and keeps them strong very beneficial for Crohn's patients.

5. Bone broths Fight inflammation. Stocks are very high in the anti-inflammatory properties including amino acids glycine and proline.

Collagen and Gelatin are the sources of bone broths immune-boosting ingredients. Collagen is the type of protein found in the connective tissue of not only humans but animals also. It's very abundant nutrient in bone marrow, cartilage and tendons. The breakdown of collagen after simmering for many hours in bone broths is what produces the gelatin. Bone broths were one of the first medicinal foods, used as medical treatments in China.

Dr Francis Pottenger a world class researcher found gelatin and collagen to have the following benefits:

- Gelatin assists people with food intolerances and sensitivities even to tolerate those foods such as cow's milk and even gluten.

- Collagen protects, soothes the lining of the intestinal tract and can assist in healing IBS, Ulcerative Colitis, Crohn's and acid reflux.

- Gelatin promotes the growth and balance of probiotics in the gut.

- Gelatin actually breaks down certain proteins and soothes the intestinal lining, proving very useful for leaky gut syndrome and healing autoimmune health problems that accompany it.

The healing Amino Acids such as gelatin in bone broths also contain a profile of amino acids like glycine, glutamine, proline and arginine. These amino acids contribute to the broths healing properties. Unfortunately, western diets are heavy on processed foods, we eat very little quality grass-fed animal products, and we are usually devoid of homemade broths, That means that our bodies are likely made deficient in these amino acid profiles and we need to consume these on a more regular basis. There are several benefits of these amino acids to our bodies especially if you're suffering from this condition.

How to make bone broth? Begin with the bones, a few pieces of the harder meats that we do not normally throw on the barbeque with fat, some vegetables, salt, pepper and some good filtered water. It's recommended to use animal parts that are not commonly found in the meat department of your local food store, parts like chicken necks, feet, knuckles, and so forth. The advantage of using chicken feet, ox feet or ox tails is that they are loaded with a tonne of connective tissues, so they make a thick gelatinous broth full of nourishing nutrients and collagen. You're best off to ask your local butcher for these parts. It's also very important to buy animal products that you know are naturally grass –fed, free of hormones and antibiotics. These free-range animals will contain far more nutrients than conventionally raised animals. These essential parts, such as the bones, fat, meat, vegetables and water make up your basic broth. Now if you're making lamb broth or beef broth, some people suggest you should brown the meat before adding it to your broth pot. Most just prefer using the raw bones. Fish and chicken can also be put directly in broth pot without browning first as well.

1. Place your bones into a large broth pot, enough that will last you for at least a week or so and cover with water.

2. Discard the first initial cooking water especially when cooking larger bones such as pig, cow or lamb. If you don't discard this water, your broth may not taste as good. When you boil these larger bones immediately blood comes out of

these raw bones, especially the pork bones. This is the reason for poor tasting broths that some may experience. If you put the heat on very low temperature and let the water slowly warm up. After about an hour or so, you will notice the water will be almost brown colour. Discard this first water.

3. Drain your bones and refill with water again. Place your lid on the back on broth pot.

4. Now you can add two tablespoons of apple cider vinegar, to your broth water prior to cooking. This step is very is extremely important and should never be missed. This helps pull out nutrients and minerals from the bones.

5. Cook very slowly over low heat. Once you see the boil begins, reduce the heat on your stove to its lowest point, so the broth slowly simmers. Approximately it should take you two hours of simmering to extract flavours and most of the gelatin from fish bones. Larger animals take slightly longer about 8-24 hours for stock made from duck, chicken or turkey. Beef broth requires the longest time 12-24 hours and if it's all mixed together just simmer for 12-24 hours

6. You will notice what I like to call scum! This will rise to the surface during cooking. What you may think or believe that this is actually fat rising to the surface, but in reality, this is actually some of the impurities, these are proteins called lectins

and other not so savoury things coming out of the parts in your lovely broth. Your broth will certainly become much tastier once you remove these elements with a spoon. This is one of the core principles of making great bone broth, is removing of the scum. Otherwise, your broth may have some funky flavours. So skim and skim some more.

7. The last step is I recommend adding onions, carrots, garlic, celery and other herbs like thyme, dill and parsley for added nutrient value and a much better flavour.

Some perfectionists will place their broth in the fridge to chill their broth and remove the fat. After putting your broth in the fridge for a few hours or overnight, you can strain the fat out. The fat will rise to the top, and then you have the option of skimming it off. I prefer leaving the fat in so it has a very nice fat source in my stock. It's your preference.

The Stock will keep well for several days in the refrigerator, or you may want it frozen in plastic containers for longer term keep. Once you place it in the refrigerator, your broth will turn into jell like substance, that's because Jell-O is actually made from gelatin – and gelatin is exactly what you got and have extracted from your bones. Great job!

Bone Broth Therapy! let's forget the couch! Have some bone broth! The collagen and other essential nutrients in the broth will heal your intestinal lining and reduce inflammation. Making you feel a whole lot better over some time of course.

How much do you consume? Well, I recommend consuming approximately 8oz (236 ml) on a daily bases as a plain beverage, or even as a light meal before you go to bed. I typically drink 8oz (236 ml) at least 4 -5 days a week for best results.

Bone broths are essential in your 90-day healing journey; broths are one of the secrets to health and long life. Science validates and has shown us that what our grandmothers knew made all the sense in the world. Bone broth is an extremely nutrient-rich food source full of healthy minerals. The stock made from bones of these animals, helps us build stronger bones ourselves, shorten recovery from colds, flu's, and is a perfect food to eat when doing intermittent fasting giving your colon a break or an even an extended fast if you need nourishment. Forget juice! If you happen to do a bone broth fast, it's loaded with more nutrients then you require during a fast. If you're also ill or nauseous, bone stocks are the perfect nourishing recovery food.

Anyone would be wise to making homemade broth as part of their regular diet. In the typical US household, homemade broths are rarer this seems to be a lost arsenal in today's world with most people opting to use premade, boxed garbage in their recipes. These boxed broths do not contain the flavour or essential nutrients and good fats of the homemade stocks.

Water: Is life! The water we put in our mouths is one of the most essential components that life itself is made up of the human body itself is made up of huge part of water, our bodies can survive for long time without food but without water we can only live a several days. Undoubtedly the greatest resource in the world. So how important is the water that we drink every day and how much of it should we drink every day?

The water we have available through most major cities in North America is highly polluted with industrial waste, sewage, mining activities, accidental oil leakage, marine dumping chemical fertilizers, pesticides, radioactive waste, medications put down the toilet, leakage from landfills and animal waste this list just can go one forever. Do you really want to drink all this crap in your water? As much as we take water in our big cities for granted; we just turn on the tap and surprise! Surprise! you have water ! How convenient. The thing is because we take water for granted and don't realize how toxic it is in our bodies it's for this reason most of the population feels we don't live in a third world country if it comes out of the tap it must therefore be clean to drink, WRONG!!

If you want to start with a healthy foundation to heal you must eat good food and drink clean water, I do not advise to drink tap water for any good reason. What are my options then? well you should be drinking filtered water is ideal however if you don't have good filtered water or can't afford a filter then only drink bottled water and if you can't afford that then at least thoroughly boil your water before you drink it.

How much water should you drink in a day? Water is a cleanser for your body it flushes away all the harmful things out of your system so the more of it you can drink to stay hydrated and to flush out your kidneys and liver then you should be drinking as much as you can. At least 4-6 10oz glasses a day should be the minimum.

"Water is the driving force of all nature"

Leonardo Da Vinci

10-Lets recap the entire program

In the previous chapter, I went over in detail what you need to do step by step. We reviewed the supplements, herbs, and what you need to eat on your 90-day program. Now it's your turn. You have made it this far, now it's time to take action. Don't procrastinate; there is no moment like now and time doesn't stop for anyone. By taking action now, in 90 days you could be healed, symptom free, feeling great, healthy, full of energy again, and having your social life back. You don't want to look back from now three months down the road being in the same situation that you are in now with your health in shambles.

Let's recap your general steps to get started.

1- Read this book thoroughly a few times if you have to, and refer to it often. Stay motivated and don't give up.

2- Be at peace with yourself and let go of all your eternal stress. Breath deep and learn to be in a relaxed state as much as possible or even practice meditation on a daily basis. Try and stay out of dramatic events.

3- Go out and buy all your supplements so you have everything to start.

4- Get yourself a journal so you can start keeping track of your program from day one. Scribble down everything you eat, when you eat it, what supplements you took, and when. And also very important, write down how many washroom trips you make, how your condition is, how you feel, your energy levels, and how your stools look for that particular day. Adjust and monitor.

5- Take hot Epson salt baths when you are in pain or bloated this really helps. Or to even de-stress.

6- Your first step should be the Liver Gallbladder cleanse so plan to start with that. Don't skip this step!

7- Start with the most basic factor of your program. Follow the SCD Diet, eat clean, and drink good clean water.

8- Start taking all your supplements and herbs vitamins and minerals. Monitor your progress and adjust accordingly. Ween off of your prescription meds as your symptoms start to disappear with your doctor's supervision.

9- Go for short walks every day when possible. Exercise stimulates the endocrine system releasing healing hormones in the body. Exercise also helps move the bowels.

10- Get as much of a good night's sleep as possible. The body only heals while you sleep or have long rest periods, so get plenty of it.

"A lot of men are afraid of settling for second best in life. But real men don't settle – instead, they step up, and decide to become the kind of man who deserves the best."

Quote by Daniel Vercetti

11-Final words

Colitis and Crohn's disease are both incredibly disruptive conditions that affect peoples' ability to hold a job, maintain social relationships, or even plan everyday events. At least for me, it totally set my life upside down in every way. Because the symptoms of these conditions are so unpredictable and painful, they often rob individuals of their ability to lead normal lives. Fortunately, by following this 90-day program outlined in this book, it can bring the soothing effects and the healing potential to treat some or all of the symptoms. My hope is to help people with Crohn's Disease and Crohn's Disease do everything from maintain a job, improve social relationships, and encourage them to live a healthier life. Empower yourself to take your health seriously and into your own hands!

I wish all of you the best of luck with your 90-day journey. Stay positive, stay strong, and don't verge and you will see great results!